Your Child and X-rays

A Parent's Guide to Radiation, X-rays and Other Imaging Procedures

Avice M. O'Connell, M. D.
and Norma Leonardi Leone

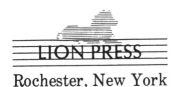

LION PRESS

Rochester, New York

YOUR CHILD AND X-RAYS

A Parent's Guide to Radiation,
X-Rays and Other Imaging Procedures.

Inquiries should be addressed to:

Lion Press
P. O. Box 92541
Rochester, NY 14692

Printed in the United States of America

X-ray Photographs by Tony Leone
Photographs by Jeffrey R. Blackman

Library of Congress Cataloging in Publication Data
O'Connell, Avice M., 1950-
    Your child and X-rays.

        Bibliography: p.
        Includes index.
        1. Pediatric radiography—Popular works.
2. X-rays—Health aspects. 3. Diagnostic imaging—
Health aspects.   I. Leone, Norma Leonardi, 1935-
II. Title
RJ51.R3026 1987   618.92'007572   87-37854
ISBN 0-936635-05-3

ii

FOR TIM AND TONY

ACKNOWLEDGMENTS

We thank our many physician friends who read some or all of the manuscript at various stages of progress and made helpful comments: Doctors Joan Furnas, Margaret Colgan, Harry Griffiths, John Colgan, Charles Lewis, B. G. Brogdon and Suzanne Klein.

We also thank Robert J. Pizzutiello, Jr., for his technical assistance.

Our thanks also go to Kate Alonzo, Don O'Connor, Nancy Howard, and Cinda and Michael Gilmore for their comments as parents.

Finally, we are deeply grateful to Jean Koenemann for her invaluable critical comments.

Contents

Introduction

Fear of radiation is natural and universal. Unfortunately, few people have a true and balanced understanding of radiation in general and X-rays in particular.

This book explains radiation in simple terms and helps to reduce the misunderstanding and fear about radiation used for medical purposes. Explanations of how much (or how little) radiation is received during various X-ray examinations puts the use of radiation into perspective with other risks of life and daily living.

Since we are unable to avoid exposure to radiation in some form, it is wise to learn about the different types of radiation and to understand the risks and benefits associated with it. A balanced look at radiation can do much to reduce fears and to help parents understand that its use is essential to the health care of their children.

CHAPTER ONE

The Radiation Story

Who's afraid of radiation? Just about everyone.
That fear is even greater when a child is involved.
But learning something about radiation—what it is,
how much is safe, how it can be helpful, and when
there is cause for concern—can do much to ease the
fears of parents whose children must have X-rays.

What follows in this and the next two chapters is
an explanation of the various forms of radiation,
with special emphasis on X-rays. Although the
information appears detailed and technical, this
detail is necessary for a more complete understanding of the information in subsequent chapters
and offers a perspective for considering the role of
X-rays in medicine and health.

The type of radiation used in medical X-rays is
electromagnetic radiation. Electromagnetic radiation
comes from many sources and in many forms other
than medical X-rays. We are constantly surrounded
by some of these forms of electromagnetic radiation,
such as cosmic radiation from space and ultraviolet
radiation from the sun. This type of radiation,
known as "background radiation," has been present
since life began.

Background radiation also includes radioactivity from minerals in the earth's crust. These minerals are commonly found in building materials that come from the earth, such as bricks, stones and cement. Very small amounts of radioactive minerals are also present in the food we eat, and tiny amounts of radiation come from television sets, computer screens and video display terminals (VDTs). In addition, radioactivity is also introduced into the atmosphere by nuclear weapons testing and occasionally by nuclear accidents. There is no fundamental difference between natural (background) radiation and man-made radiation.

Other forms of electromagnetic radiation include visible light, infrared radiation, radio waves and microwaves. Most forms of radiation, not just X-rays, can be dangerous in their own way if misused. For example, excessive exposure to sunlight can cause sunburn, premature aging of the skin and even skin cancer years later. Microwaves and infrared waves that are so useful for cooking and heating can severely burn and damage human tissue if used without regard for normal safety precautions. Constant exposure to visible light can upset some natural body rhythms, such as sleep patterns.

Although there are many similarities among the various types of radiation, there are also major differences. All types of radiation are alike in that they are all forms of energy and all have a wave form or configuration. In addition, all types of electromagnetic radiation travel at the speed of light. But the various types of radiation differ in the length of their waves, or wavelengths, which can vary from miles to millionths of a centimeter. The length of their waves determines their effect on the body.

The Electromagnetic Spectrum

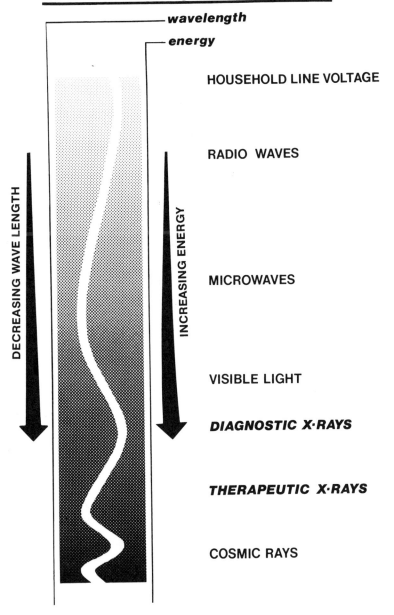

The longest waves are electric and radio waves; the shortest are gamma and cosmic rays. As wavelengths become shorter their energy levels rise, and this is what allows X-rays, gamma and cosmic rays to penetrate substances to varying degrees, depending upon the physical composition of the substance. Living body tissues such as skin, muscle and lungs are easily penetrated, whereas bone is not. Non-living materials such as plastic and wood are also easily penetrated, but concrete and lead are not.

High energy waves, or rays, are called *ionizing radiation*. In very high doses, they can produce harmful effects on living cells. There is, however, no evidence that they produce harmful effects in very small doses. Scientists cannot say that there are absolutely no effects from small amounts of ionizing radiation; they can say only that the effects are so small that they are undetectable and produce no change in the function or growth of the human body.

Because of their short wavelength and thus their ability to penetrate the body, X-rays can be used to form an image of the internal structure of the body on film. These images provide doctors with valuable information that cannot be obtained as safely or as easily in any other way. Diagnostic X-rays cannot be felt as they pass through the body, since they cause no heat, pain or any other sensation.

X-rays have been in use since 1895, when they were discovered by Wilhelm Conrad Roentgen. Roentgen was awarded the first Nobel Prize for Physics for his discovery, which launched the age of modern physics and resulted in major changes in the practice of medicine.

Diagnostic X-rays have now been used for more than 90 years, and during this time doctors and other scientists have learned much about the safest and most effective ways to use them. Modern X-ray equipment and film use the lowest doses of radiation possible and yet provide the sharpest images ever. When X-rays are used for medical purposes, radiation is used in small, precisely controlled amounts.

Radiation from medical X-rays can be compared to the use of many other common elements, such as fire and electricity. For example, fire can cause terrible destruction when it rages out of control. But when used in controlled amounts, it can also provide heat for survival, comfort and cooking. Similarly, electricity can be dangerous and damaging, as seen in occasional unfortunate accidents involving high tension electrical power lines or the "natural" source, lightning. When used carefully, however, electricity is used daily by all of us, including children, to provide light and energy for many of our necessities at home, school and work.

Radiation in extremely large amounts can also cause death and destruction of the type that occurred after the bombing of Hiroshima and Nagasaki and the Chernobyl nuclear reactor accident. But in medical diagnostic X-rays, radiation is used in small, calculated amounts and provides valuable information to help a doctor make or exclude a diagnosis (the information from a negative examination can be just as important as that from a positive one).

With the information obtained from medical X-rays, doctors are able to detect injury, disease and other abnormalities in their early stages. When medical problems or diseases are diagnosed early, any needed treatment can begin promptly, and early recovery is much more likely. Early diagnosis

and treatment benefit both the child and the parents
and contribute to good health care today.

CHAPTER TWO

Effects of Radiation on the Body

When people think of the dangers of radiation, they naturally remember the major radiation disasters and their consequences. The dangers of diagnostic levels of radiation, however, are very small when compared with those from nuclear explosions and nuclear reactor accidents. A nuclear explosion or nuclear power plant accident produces radiation levels that are hundreds or thousands of times the levels used in diagnostic X-rays. There is no easy way to compare these massive doses with the amount of radiation used in medical X-rays.

Scientists and mathematicians have tried to calculate the true dangers from diagnostic X-rays. They take the effects of the enormous amounts of radiation, such as those from the atomic bomb explosions, and try to scale them down to the relatively tiny amounts used in diagnostic X-ray examinations. There is no way to tell if these are accurate calculations because they cannot be proved.

In order to prove these calculations scientifically, thousands of people would have to be exposed to known doses of radiation and then followed for their lifetimes to detect any increased numbers of cancers or leukemia over the normal rate in the population. Similarly, in order to prove the calculations of genetic defects, future generations would have to be studied. This type of experiment would be impossible to set up, since it would be unethical to expose anyone to radiation for experimental purposes.

Scientists do the best they can by using fruit flies and mice for experiments, but they cannot say that the effects are definitely the same in humans. There may even be a level of radiation below which there is absolutely no danger, but scientists do not know whether the result of radiation is always directly proportional to the dose (for example, half the dose gives half the effect).

Apart from the lethal effects of extremely high doses of radiation, there are three possible major effects of radiation on the human body: cancer, genetic changes, and congenital abnormalities. But any of these effects is also very difficult to prove in a given situation. Diseases caused by radiation do not look any different from naturally occurring diseases. We all have an approximately 30% lifetime risk of cancer already, regardless of radiation exposure.[1]

Similarly, it would be very difficult to connect problems in pregnancy and birth defects with radiation, since as many as 25% of early pregnancies miscarry, for many and often unexplained reasons. In addition, 5% of all live born babies have some congenital abnormality, so that a slight increase resulting from diagnostic X-rays would be very difficult to prove in a given situation.

[1] American Cancer Society, Cancer Facts and Figures-1988 (New York, NY, 1988).

Most of the radiation received by the human body comes from natural sources. (See chart, below.)

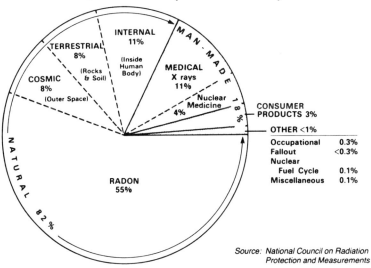

Sources of Radiation Exposure to U.S. Population

Occupational	0.3%
Fallout	<0.3%
Nuclear	
Fuel Cycle	0.1%
Miscellaneous	0.1%

Source: *National Council on Radiation Protection and Measurements*

The entire population receives more than 80% of its radiation from natural sources in the earth, air and water. Only 15% comes from medical X-rays, X-ray therapy and nuclear medicine. The other 5% or less comes from a combination of nuclear weapons testing, nuclear power and occupational exposure.

We do not see or feel the natural, or background, radiation that is always around us and has always been present. Most people are unaware of its presence. Similarly, we cannot see or feel diagnostic radiation.

Even though we cannot see or feel radiation, there is much concern about what happens when radiation from any source reaches the human body. When radiation reaches the human body, some is absorbed by the skin and some by the tissues inside. For diagnostic X-rays, the amount of radiation used must be enough to pass through the body and expose a film so that an X-ray image is formed. As it passes through, some radiation from the X-rays is absorbed by the cells which form the body.

In order to understand the effects of radiation on the human body, it is helpful to understand something about the radiation used and the basic cellular structure of the human body. X-rays are called *ionizing radiation* because when they are absorbed in the body, they may displace an electron from an atom to form an ion. Electrons, along with protons and neutrons, make up the structure of an atom. Atoms grouped together form molecules, and combinations of different molecules form the cells which make up the many different tissues of the body.

When radiation strikes a cell, it causes one of several reactions: 1) It may pass through without doing any damage at all. 2) An ion may be formed. Even if an ion is formed, it may cause no lasting effect. 3) If many ions are formed, a cell may be damaged. Since some cells are more sensitive than others, a damaged cell may be repaired or replaced by the body, depending upon the type of cell affected. 4) A cell may be damaged beyond repair.

The effect of damaged cells on the whole body depends on which cells are affected and whether or not they can be replaced. The degree of overall damage will depend on how much radiation is received and how much or what parts of the body are involved.

The problems of estimating and comparing the consequences of enormous amounts of radiation exposure to the very low levels of radiation used in diagnostic radiology make it extremely difficult to draw any scientific conclusions about low doses of radiation. In an atomic bomb explosion or a nuclear reactor accident, the whole body receives radiation. But when radiation is used for medical purposes such as X-rays, the amount of the body exposed is specifically defined and the amount of radiation is carefully calculated.

Scientists continue to study the effects of radiation on the body, but these effects remain difficult to prove. We do know, however, that it has never been shown conclusively that any significant damage occurs to the human body at the levels of radiation used in diagnostic radiology.

CHAPTER THREE
How Much Radiation is Safe?

People ask how much radiation is safe, how much is too much, and what can be done to control the amount used. Is there a number which, when exceeded, causes danger to life or future generations? There are no easy answers. Remember, radiation is not a modern creation, and natural radiation far exceeds man-made sources of radiation.

More than half the natural radiation comes from radon, a radioactive gas which results from the decay of uranium, which is a radioactive mineral in the earth's crust. Radon is a colorless, odorless gas which is present in varying amounts in the ground around and beneath our homes and in building materials such as brick and concrete.

The rest of the natural radiation exposure we receive comes from *cosmic* radiation from outer space, *terrestrial* radiation which is in rocks and soil and *internal* radiation from inside our own bodies. The source of internal radiation is the food we eat and the milk and water we drink. The radiation in our food and drink comes from water, plants, and animals which receive radiation from the earth.

Within the United States and from country to country across the world, there is also a wide variation in background, or natural, radiation. This is because of geographical differences in altitude and differences in the composition of the earth and minerals in each country.

For example, the annual background radiation in Florida is half the annual background radiation in Denver, Colorado. This difference is because Florida is at sea level, and Denver is at a high altitude. The earth's atmosphere filters cosmic rays, so that the higher one goes above sea level, the greater the cosmic radiation level. This is also why flying contributes a small amount of radiation. Flying at the common altitude of 33,000 feet or more removes some of the screening effect of the atmosphere.

Around the world, there is a wide variation in background radiation because of differing amounts of naturally occurring radiation in the earth's crust. For example, the background radiation in France is twice the United States'average, and parts of India have ten times the U. S. amount. *Even with all this variation in background radiation, however, no increase in the incidence in cancer or congenital abnormalities has been detected in these areas.*

In addition to the background radiation, approximately 5% of the annual radiation exposure to the population of the United States comes from a combination of nuclear weapons testing, the nuclear fuel industry and occupational exposure in medicine and in industry.

One other source of radiation which has recently been recognized is cigarette smoke. Smokers receive an additional dose of radiation to their lungs from a radioactive material called polonium, which is released in the burning of tobacco. Unfortunately, non-smokers inhaling cigarette smoke may also receive some radiation from smoke. So you can see that there are many and often unrecognized sources of radiation all around us every day.

Medical X-rays account for about 15% of the annual radiation exposure in the United States. This figure includes the radiation used in radiation therapy and in nuclear medicine.

Medical radiation is, of course, used by choice. The doctor ordering the X-ray has a question or concern that can best be answered by an X-ray examination. X-rays are now commonly used to help in the early diagnosis of many diseases and injuries. Depending upon the severity of the problem, the number and complexity of X-ray examinations needed to diagnose and determine the extent of an illness or problem increase.

Even with multiple and repeated X-ray examinations, however, the total dose will still be hundreds or thousands of times less than the exposure of many Japanese to the radiation from the bombs at the end of World War II. Remember also that during a medical X-ray examination, only a specific part of the body is examined, whereas the whole body is exposed during a radiation accident or an atomic explosion.

In spite of the safety of medical X-rays, however, the expected benefits of the X-rays must always outweigh any possible risk in order for the examination to be performed. In the days before the discovery of X-rays, some diseases were not diagnosed as early as they are now and were often far advanced at the time they were diagnosed. In the years before X-rays were used, many more people died of undetected infections, injuries, cancers and other diseases. People tend to be more concerned about radiation risks than other hazards of daily life, but in reality there are many risks greater than those from radiation. Figures have been developed which compare the risks of radiation with other risks of daily life, as shown in the following table.[2]

INDIVIDUAL ACTION	MINUTES OF LIFE EXPECTANCY LOST
Calorie-rich dessert	50
Non-diet soft drink	15
Not fastening seat belt	0.1/mile
Smoking a cigarette	10
Coast-to-coast flight	100
Coast-to-coast drive	1000
1 mrem of radiation	1.5

The unit of radiation used in this table is a *millirem*, which is one thousandth of a rem. *Rads* and *rems* are units of absorbed dose of radiation. The rem includes a factor which relates specifically to the effect of the radiation on the human body. Rad stands for *radiation absorbed dose* and rem stands for *radiation equivalent (in) man*. For diagnostic X-rays, one rad equals one rem. These terms are still used to express radiation dosages, although new international units called *Grays* and *Sieverts* are now being adopted. One Gray is equivalent to 100 rads, and one Sievert is 100 rems.

In these calculations, one millirem (one thousandth of a rem) of radiation reduces life expectancy 1.5 minutes, which is much safer than smoking cigarettes, eating rich desserts and driving

[2] Bernard L. Cohen and I-Sing Lee, "A Catalog of Risks," Health Physics, Vol. 36 (June 1979) p. 721.

long distances, especially without a seat belt. A single chest X-ray is as potentially dangerous as driving 5 miles on the highway or smoking two cigarettes. Many people accept the risks of these activities, and many are unaware that these risks exist. The radiation in a necessary diagnostic X-ray examination is a relatively minor risk in comparison.

Information on the risks from low levels of ionizing radiation is available from studies by an advisory committee to the National Academy of Sciences. Their report is called "The Biological Effects of Ionizing Radiation," or the BEIR report.[3]

To give some idea of the actual radiation dose of a diagnostic X-ray examination, a chest X-ray can be used as an example. Remember, however, that in all diagnostic X-ray examinations, the dose depends upon the size of the patient as well as on the type of examination.

A single view from the front of the chest of a person who measures nine inches from front to back (through the center of the chest) results in a very small dose of radiation, usually under 15 millirems. This is the dose received by the skin, which is considerably more than the dose received by the center of the chest. The skin dose is the usual measurement given when radiation doses are calculated, but a more accurate measurement, if possible, would be one taken inside, at the center of the chest. It is very difficult to give an exact measurement of the true radiation to a given person without knowing all the details of that person's size as well as the type of examination being performed. This is why there is no simple answer to the question parents often ask regarding the exact radiation dose

[3]Report of the Committee on Biological Effects of Ionizing Radiation. National Academy Press, 1980.

a child will receive from a specific examination. X-ray examinations are tailored to each child's size and are also modified as needed, depending upon the nature of the problem being investigated.

Responsible parents surely try their best to minimize risks to themselves and to their children, but realize that life cannot be totally free of risks— or radiation. In order to minimize the risk of any possible harmful effects from radiation, parents can take some precautions regarding their own health and that of their children when X-rays are concerned.

One important precaution is to be sure that X-rays are taken *only* on the recommendation of a qualified physician. A physician is able to balance the benefits of having the X-ray exam against the risk of causing any possible side effects.

If a physician recommends an X-ray examination, parents may want to ask him or her about the type of information expected from this examination, whether or not an X-ray is the best way to obtain that information, and how the care of the child will be affected by the results of the examination.

X-rays should always be taken on up-to-date, well maintained equipment. The Food and Drug Administration has strict standards for the manufacture and installation of all X-ray equipment, and individual states have specific regulations for the registration and maintenance of an X-ray facility. A certificate noting registration by the State Health Department Bureau of Radiation Safety or similar licensing agency should be posted in all offices where any type of X-rays are taken. Annual inspection ensures that the equipment and procedures are in continual compliance with these standards. Many X-ray offices and hospitals have detailed programs for continued quality and safety of performance.

In addition to the use of properly maintained equipment, it is also important that the personnel using the equipment be trained and qualified to use it. The person who actually takes the X-ray is usually a radiologic technologist or radiographer. Radiologic technologists or radiographers have had two or more years of training in the use of X-rays. In some states, they are certified by the state, and these states require that a registration certificate for technologists be posted in all departments and offices where X-rays are taken. Regulations for technologists vary from state to state. There is a National Registry for Radiologic Technologists, and some states require a technologist to pass the Registry examination in order to obtain a license to practice in that state.

After the X-rays are taken, they must be interpreted (or "read") by someone trained to understand what is seen on the film. Although some doctors who are not radiologists have X-ray equipment in their offices so they can take and interpret their own X-rays, most doctors prefer to send their patients to an X-ray office and have the films interpreted by a radiologist. X-rays that are taken in an emergency room are usually read initially by the doctor ordering them and then reviewed later by a radiologist.

All doctors receive some training in the interpretation of X-rays, but radiologists are specialists in the use of X-rays in medicine. A radiologist is a medical doctor who has had an additional three or more years of education and training in the use of diagnostic X-rays and other imaging procedures and in interpreting X-rays. Radiologists who receive this training and pass strict examinations after completion of their training are certified by the American College of Radiology, the national educational and professional board for radiologists in the United States.

You may wonder how people who work with X-rays all day long are affected by the radiation they use constantly. Part of the training for radiologic technologists and radiologists is to learn safety rules for working with X-ray equipment. There is a formula for acceptable annual and lifetime levels of radiation for people who work with X-rays. These people wear radiation-detection badges which monitor the amount of radiation to which they are exposed.

In the early days after the discovery of X-rays, the dangers of excessive radiation were not recognized. But now, safety procedures have been established for more than 70 years. By following these procedures to regulate their exposure, radiologists and radiologic technologists are as likely as the general population to live long and healthy lives and to have normal, healthy children. They do not, as a group, have any increased risk of cancer or leukemia, and they have the same life expectancy as people with similar occupations who do not use radiation.

CHAPTER FOUR

Diagnostic X-rays

The terms "diagnostic X-rays" or "diagnostic radiology" describe the use of X-rays to help diagnose suspected health problems. X-rays provide doctors with a way to "see" what is going on inside the body. X-rays are used to visualize bones, joints, organs such as the heart, brain, lungs, stomach, kidneys, bladder, and just about any other part of the body.

When more information is needed to help with diagnosis or treatment, a doctor will often request that a child have diagnostic X-rays. Diagnostic X-rays are carefully controlled and specifically directed at an area of concern, such as the chest, spine, finger, and so forth. The whole body does NOT receive radiation—only the specific area which is being examined (see illustration). As an additional precaution, lead shielding may be used to cover other parts of the body. (The use of shielding is described more completely in Chapter 8.)

The actual time of the average X-ray exposure is extremely short: often much less than one second. Some of the radiation penetrates the part of the patient's body being examined, and this creates the X-ray image. The remainder of the radiation is absorbed and dispersed immediately by the body, but the amount is so small that any damage is extremely unlikely.

When an X-ray is taken, the part of the body to be examined is placed between the X-ray tube (camera) and the unexposed film. The patient stands, sits, or lies down, depending on the examination being performed. The X-ray beam passes through the area of the body being examined to reach the film. The film is held in a flat, light-tight (or light-sealed) box called a *cassette*.

The film is sandwiched between two *intensifying screens*. These screens are called intensifying because they increase, or strengthen, the effect of the X-ray alone. The screens contain crystals which are stimulated by an X-ray and give off light. This in turn forms an image on the film, adding to and increasing the image formed by the X-ray itself. The use of screens dramatically reduces the amount of radiation needed to form an image. Without intensifying screens, a radiation dose of 50 to 100 times more would be necessary for the same image.

The special type of film used in X-rays is also highly sensitive to the small amounts of radiation and the small amounts of light from the intensifying screens. This film allows further reduction in the amount of radiation used to perform an X-ray examination.

In order to understand what happens when an X-ray is taken, a comparison can be made with the use of a camera in taking a photograph. The X-ray exposes the film to form an image, just as light exposes the film inside a camera. The film in a camera is then developed and used to make a photographic print, or it is used directly as a slide and viewed with transmitted light. The X-ray film is also developed, and it is viewed with transmitted light on a lighted box.

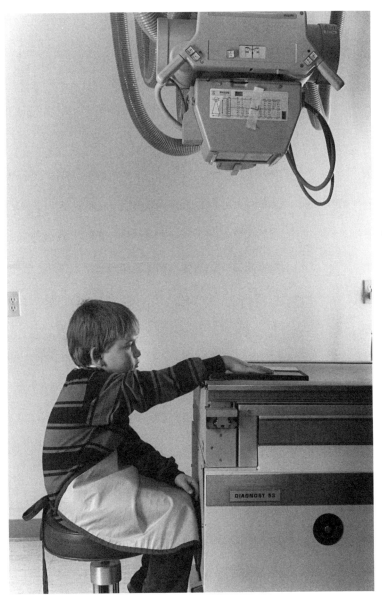

Child ready for X-ray of hand or wrist. For this type of examination, hand is placed directly on film cassette. Note lead apron shielding lower part of body.

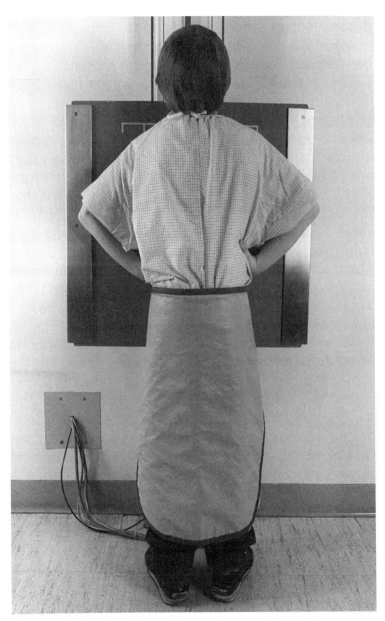

Child ready for chest X-ray. Note lead apron shielding lower part of body.

The X-ray image on the film is white, black and shades of grey, depending upon the composition of the part of the body it passes through. Bones are very dense because of their calcium content, so they absorb most of the X-ray beam and appear very light or white on the film. Fractures (breaks), cysts or tumors within the bone usually appear as black lines or spaces. On the other hand, lungs appear mostly black on X-ray film. This is because lungs are filled with air, which absorbs very little of the X-ray beam passing through them (to be sure that the lungs are well filled with air, patients who have chest X-rays are asked to take a deep breath and hold it while the X-ray is taken). On a chest X-ray, diseases such as pneumonia or tumors appear white against the dark background of a normal lung. If the lungs are not fully inflated, these abnormalities will not be as easily visible.

After the X-ray has been taken, the radiation is immediately absorbed in the body, and no radiation comes from the body. The process of taking an X-ray is similar to illuminating an object with a flashlight: when the light is turned off, the effect ends immediately and the object does not retain any of the light. In the same manner, when the X-ray source is turned off, all the X-rays cease, and no part of the body retains any lasting radiation or becomes radioactive. Also, no radiation is retained in the room in which the X-rays are taken, in the X-ray machine, or in the X-ray film.

Medical X-rays are used in many ways to help both the doctor and the patient. A typical example is the use of X-rays to help diagnose fractures or pneumonia. Sprains and fractures can look alike on physical examination, but an X-ray can show whether

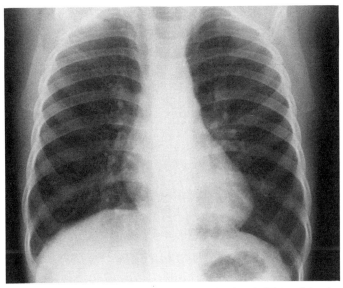

Frontal view of normal chest (called PA view). Note clear lungs (large paired dark areas).

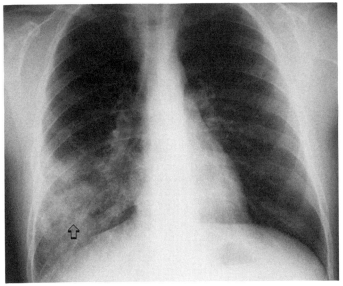

Frontal view of chest showing whitish patch (arrow), which is a pneumonia.

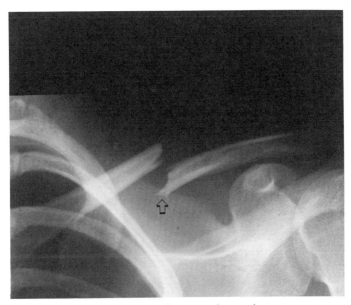

Collarbone (clavicle) showing fracture (arrow).

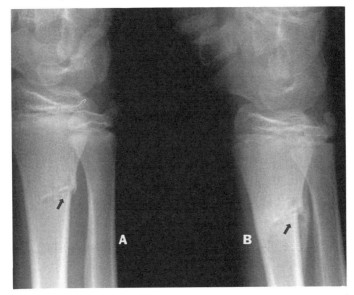

Wrist and lower forearm: A) view immediately following fracture. B) view two weeks later showing beginning of healing process.

the injury is a fracture or a sprain. A sprain cannot be "seen" on an X-ray, but if no fracture is present, a sprain is a likely cause of the problem. If there is an obvious fracture, the X-ray will show the exact location and the extent of the injury. This information guides the doctor in the correct course of treatment. Occasionally, a hairline fracture does not show immediately, and a follow-up X-ray is performed one or two weeks later.

Another common use of X-rays is to detect pneumonia. Every child who has a cough and fever does not need an X-ray. But there are many causes of fever and cough in children, and a chest X-ray can be a very important test to find out if the fever is caused by pneumonia. Pneumonia may be very difficult to diagnose by physical examination alone, especially in small children. If the doctor has to wait until the physical signs become very obvious, a child could be much more seriously ill and take longer to recover. The chest X-ray can sometimes detect pneumonia at an early stage, before there are physical signs, so that specific treatment can begin.

Although X-rays are most often used to detect disease or injury, they can also be used in cases of suspected congenital defects and accelerated or delayed bone growth ("bone age"), which may be important in evaluating a child's growth. X-rays are also used to detect and measure scoliosis (curvature of the spine), and to detect various bone or joint abnormalities, such as congenital hip dislocation, tumors and infections. These uses for X-rays are described in detail in Chapter 5.

CHAPTER FIVE

Other Common Uses of X-rays

Although the most common types of X-rays for children are chest X-rays to check for pneumonia and bone X-rays to check for fractures, there are other situations in which X-rays can greatly help in diagnosis and treatment. The following problems can often be diagnosed with some form of X-ray or imaging procedure.

SCOLIOSIS

Scoliosis is a curvature of the spine. Signs of an early curvature are often found during a school screening or routine physical examination. If the signs are severe enough on physical examination, they need to be confirmed and measured by an X-ray examination. X-rays of the spine, from the chest to the pelvis, are needed for this purpose. These X-rays may have to be repeated at a later date if the curve progresses and also to see if a brace or surgical treatment is required to prevent further deformity.

When X-rays are taken for scoliosis, special shielding techniques are used to minimize the radiation dose to the breasts of young girls. This shielding is used because the developing breasts of young girls are especially sensitive to radiation, so every effort is made to further reduce the radiation dose to this area.

BONE AGE

When a child is short or tall for his or her age, an X-ray can determine whether or not the child's bone age is close to the chronological (real) age of the child or if the bone maturity is delayed. Bone age can determine which children need further tests to evaluate the cause of their growth problem.

The bone age examination involves a single X-ray view of the child's left wrist and hand. This X-ray is compared with standards derived from X-rays of more than a thousand children, and a bone age is then determined. If the bone age is significantly less than the chronological age of the child, a catch-up period can be expected once the cause has been established and any required treatment started. If the bone age matches the chronological age, the child may remain small. Children's growth patterns, however, are extremely variable and often genetically determined. Some children may do most of their growing much later than all of their friends.

LIMP

A doctor will usually order X-rays if a child develops a limp. The limp may indicate an injury or an inflammation in the hip or other joint in the leg. A mild hip inflammation, which is a common cause of a limp, most often resolves with bed rest, but occasionally develops into a more serious condition

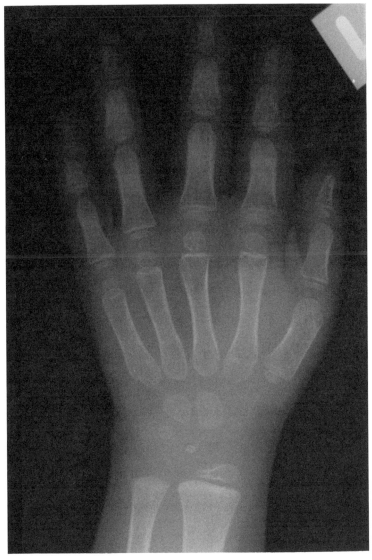

Normal hand and wrist used for bone age determination.
Above X-ray shows early development of bones in a young
child.

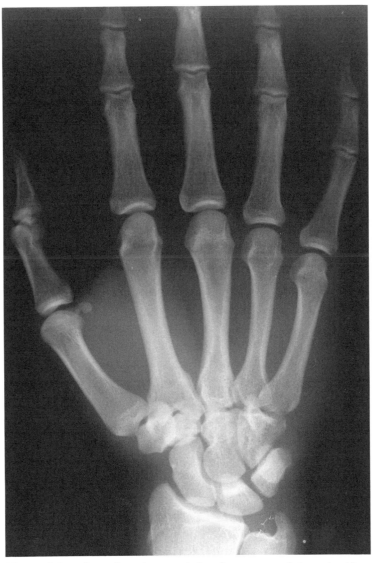

Normal hand and wrist used for bone age determination. Above X-ray shows normal development of bones in an older child.

which can damage the joint. X-rays are needed to see if a painful joint shows any signs of a more serious condition. Careful clinical, and sometimes X-ray, follow-up is often needed in these cases.

"CLICKING HIPS"

Some babies, most often girls, have "clicking" hips. This condition is usually discovered during a routine examination by a doctor. "Clicking" hips are very common and often disappear without any treatment. But if there is an abnormal physical examination of the hip which suggests possible congenital dislocation of the hip (CDH), an X-ray may be ordered. Some imaging centers use ultrasound to examine the hips of a newborn child for dislocation. This condition is initially treated by splinting the hips in the correct position to allow normal development of the joint. The splinting can be done with extra diapers, or a cast may be required. Follow-up X-rays are needed to check the position and development of the hip.

DENTAL CARE

The American Academy of Pediatric Dentists does not recommend routine dental X-rays for children. There are guidelines for the use of X-rays in pediatric dentistry, and these are very conservative. Dental X-rays of children may be taken, however, to check the number or direction of a child's permanent teeth or when needed to study a specific tooth or problem. The dose used for dental X-rays in children is quite small and is limited to a small area of the body (the mouth). When dental

X-rays are taken, a lead apron should be used to cover the rest of the child's body, and an additional lead collar may also be provided to cover the thyroid. (See explanation of the use of lead for shielding in Chapter 8).

APPENDICITIS

The diagnosis of appendicitis can be one of the most difficult diagnoses to make. Sometimes, however, it can be very easy, depending upon the individual circumstances. When a child has severe abdominal pain and is vomiting, one of the many possible causes is appendicitis. Unfortunately, there is no single easy test to help when all the typical signs and symptoms are not present. Sometimes an X-ray or an ultrasound examination of the abdomen may help in diagnosis of the problem. But physical examination, white cell count and urinalysis, combined with careful observation and follow-up, are the usual ways the diagnosis is made.

CHAPTER SIX

Contrast Examinations

Many children will have no X-rays at all during their childhood years, and others will have X-rays only for injuries or for relatively minor childhood illnesses. Some children, however, will need tests that require more complex X-ray procedures. These X-ray procedures are performed either by or under the supervision of a radiologist.

For some of these tests, doctors need to "look" at parts of the body such as the stomach or kidneys, which normally do not stand out well enough from the surrounding structures to show up on the X-ray picture. *Contrast* materials are needed to make these parts of the body more visible.

Contrast materials are liquid substances especially developed to be introduced into the body to make a particular area of the body visible on X-rays. One main group of contrast materials contains a form of iodine, often called iodine "dyes." This iodine is *not* the kind used on minor skin injuries. Some iodine "dyes" are injected into veins, some are injected into arteries, and others are introduced directly into an area of concern, such as the bladder. The other main group of contrast materials is the barium compounds. These are taken by mouth or given by enema.

Contrast examinations are common tests and may be needed if a child has frequent urinary tract infections, persistent abdominal or other pain, bleeding, weight loss, chronic diarrhea or constipation, or some other symptoms that indicate a possible medical problem.

Although some contrast examinations may be temporarily uncomfortable or unpleasant, parents and children should understand that the discomfort lasts only a few minutes. Although the discomfort may seem to last forever, the actual time for most examinations is quite short. The doctor and the technologists try to make the child as comfortable as possible during these examinations, but the nature of some procedures makes them unpleasant and sometimes even painful for a short time. A simple explanation of the procedure will often help a child to understand and accept the temporary discomfort involved. It may also help to remember that the information provided by these examinations is important for accurate diagnosis and treatment and is not easily obtained by any other means.

Children do not usually experience any aftereffects from contrast procedures. The iodine "dyes" occasionally cause reactions in adults, but very rarely in children. Reactions include hives, sneezing, or wheezing, but occasionally more serious reactions occur. A new family of "iodine dyes" has been developed and is being used increasingly. These new contrast liquids have an even lower risk of causing reactions. The other category of contrast material, barium, is a non-reactive substance and usually passes harmlessly out of the body.

Some form of contrast material is essential in all of the following examinations.

INTRAVENOUS PYELOGRAM (IVP)

An intravenous pyelogram is done to examine the structure and function of the kidneys to see if a congenital (that is, present since birth) abnormality, obstruction, scarring or tumor is present and to check normal growth and function. During an IVP, the radiologist injects contrast material (the iodine-containing liquid) into a vein, usually at the front of the elbow. A small needle is used (similar to the type used for blood tests), and the contrast itself cannot be felt. The contrast liquid is then filtered almost immediately through the kidneys, into the ureters and then into the bladder, all within minutes of the injection. X-rays are taken during the examination to show the kidneys, ureters and bladder at different stages of filtration and from various angles.

VOIDING CYSTOURETHROGRAM (VCU)

During a voiding cystourethrogram, the bladder is filled with contrast material to see if any reverse flow (called reflux) occurs from the bladder into the ureters (the drainage tubes from the kidneys). Checking for reversed flow is important because the flow should be one way only:down from the kidneys, through the ureters and into the bladder. Reflux, often associated with infections, can damage the kidneys and cause scarring and poor function years later. In addition, the VCU will check the ability of the child's bladder to empty properly and will also show any abnormalities of the urethra (the final channel from the bladder to the skin surface).

A VCU is commonly performed after the first urinary tract infection in children. Urinary tract infections are much more common in girls because they have a short urethra, which allows the bladder to be more easily infected from the outside. A urinary tract infection is less common in boys, so it is more likely to indicate some type of structural abnormality.

A VCU is a sterile (that is, clean or free of contamination) procedure. During the procedure, a nurse or trained technologist inserts a small catheter into the bladder. The catheter is a tiny, round-tipped soft plastic or rubber tube that is much smaller than the urethral opening. The area of skin around the urethral opening is first cleansed with an antiseptic solution, and the tube is then slipped into the bladder. The catheter is then taped to the leg so it will not slip out.

This procedure may cause some discomfort during the passage of the catheter, especially in boys, since the urethra is much longer than in girls. Very young children often fuss during a VCU because they do not like to be restrained. Sedation is rarely needed, especially if the child is well prepared for the examination by the parent, who must be both encouraging to the child and at the same time cooperative with the doctor and technologist performing the examination.

When the catheter is in the bladder, the contrast material is allowed to flow into the bladder until it is full (this usually takes a pint of liquid or more). The child then urinates (voids) into a pad or towels, and several X-rays of the urethra, bladder and ureters are taken, depending on what is seen on the TV monitor while the child voids. The iodine is expelled painlessly and unnoticed in the urine. Sometimes, however, children experience slight discomfort on voiding for several voidings after the procedure.

GALLBLADDER SERIES

A gallbladder series is rarely performed on children. This procedure is also a contrast examination, used to detect gallbladder abnormalities, such as stones. The contrast is given in the form of tablets which are taken on the night before the examination. The contrast material used for a gallbladder series often causes diarrhea.

If there is a need to examine a child's gallbladder, the doctor will often recommend an ultrasound examination, which does not require the use of ionizing radiation or the use of any contrast material.

ARTHROGRAM

An arthrogram is an X-ray examination of a joint, most commonly the knee joint. In order to see the joint surfaces and outline the ligaments and cartilage, contrast material is needed. Contrast material similar to the type used for an IVP is injected into the joint, along with some air, and then a series of X-ray pictures are taken from various angles.

The examination begins with an injection of a local anesthetic similar to the type used by dentists. Then a small needle is inserted into the joint, and the contrast material and air are injected. The air, along with the contrast material, helps to outline the ligaments and cartilage inside the knee joint, so that any tear or broken fragment can be seen.

Air causes a strange feeling because the joint becomes distended and is under pressure. This creates a feeling similar to having a lot of fluid in the knee, as often happens after an injury. After an arthrogram, there is usually some discomfort, which may last for several days.

Usual candidates for arthrograms are athletic boys and girls involved in contact sports. The examination is commonly ordered by an orthopedic surgeon. During an arthrogram, the radiation is directed only at the knee or whatever joint is being examined.

ANGIOCARDIOGRAM

Occasionally, children are born with abnormalities of the heart and major blood vessels. In the past, these abnormalities were evaluated by an angiocardiogram, which is an X-ray examination of the heart and surrounding blood vessels entering and leaving it. Congenital cardiac abnormalities are now commonly evaluated by an *echocardiogram*, which is an "echo," or ultrasound, examination of all the chambers of the heart and the large veins and arteries entering and leaving it (see Chapter 7 for an explanation of ultrasound examinations).

The kinds of abnormalities which may be present are various blockages and abnormal connections or holes between some of the chambers of the heart. These abnormalities interfere with the normal direction and flow of blood through the heart and lungs.

ANGIOGRAM

An angiogram is rarely performed on children. The procedure involves the injection of contrast ("dye") into an artery (this is also called an arteriogram) or into a vein (this is also called a venogram).Some examples of angiograms are a cerebral angiogram, which examines the blood vessels of the brain, and a renal angiogram, which examines the blood vessels of the kidney.

BARIUM EXAMINATIONS

Barium is used to examine the gastrointestinal (GI) tract. Barium is a natural substance which is present in the earth. It is mined and then processed into the form (barium sulphate) used for X-ray examinations. Barium is safe and does not dissolve or react in the body. It is useful as a contrast material because it blocks the path of an X-ray beam, thereby making an area (such as the stomach) appear white against a dark background. Iodine and calcium (a natural contrast material in the body) do the same, as do lead and concrete, which are used for protection and shielding from X-rays.

Barium sulphate is a powder, which is mixed with water so that it can be swallowed or given as a enema. Barium is used in all of the following examinations:

UPPER GI SERIES (UGI)

During an upper GI examination, the patient drinks the barium (usually about 1/2 to 2 cups, depending upon the size of the child and the nature of the problem). The barium is mixed into a chalky-tasting liquid that is like a thick milk shake in consistency (but not in taste) and may be pink and strawberry flavored. Babies and small children can be given the barium from a baby bottle. Tiny babies who are too small or too sick to suck may be given barium through a very small feeding tube.

Older children may be given effervescent liquids or small crystals to drink before the barium. The liquids or crystals make a gas (carbon dioxide), which distends the stomach for better detail of the lining of the esophagus, stomach and duodenum. During the GI series, the radiologist watches the barium as it travels through the GI tract. This is done with a *fluoroscope*, which is like an X-ray video camera. The fluoroscope is moved over the patient as needed and produces an image of the GI tract on a television monitor. The examination may also be videotaped for review or to demonstrate any abnormalities to the referring doctor.

The esophagus, stomach and duodenum are examined as the barium passes down through the upper part of the GI tract. The esophagus is the narrow muscular tube leading from the mouth to the stomach; the duodenum comes after the stomach and is the first part of the small bowel. A GI series only takes a few minutes once the barium is swallowed. While the radiologist watches the barium flow through the stomach, he or she takes spot (still) films of any areas of interest. The technologist then takes overhead films. These are a standardized series of pictures which include the entire stomach and duodenum in different views, taken with an overhead X-ray tube (camera).

If the small bowel (small intestine) is also to be examined, then, following the UGI, the patient is given more barium to drink. This procedure is called a small bowel *follow-through*. Films are taken every half hour until the barium has passed through the entire small bowel (which can be as long as 30 feet). This usually takes 30 to 60 minutes, but may take as much as two to four hours.

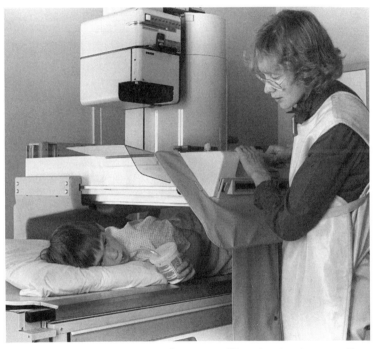

Child ready to drink barium for upper GI series, barium swallow or small bowel series. Radiologist is positioning fluoroscope over child.

BARIUM SWALLOW or ESOPHAGRAM

A barium swallow or esophagram is an examination of the swallowing mechanism and the esophagus. The same form of barium that is used for the upper GI series is used for this examination. In fact, an esophagram is most often combined with the upper GI series as one examination.

BARIUM ENEMA

A barium enema is an examination of the large bowel (the colon or large intestine), performed when ulceration, inflammation, obstruction or a tumor is suspected. As the name states, it is an enema, using barium. The enema tube is plastic, with a rounded tip, and is connected to the bag of barium. The radiologist often uses a hand pump to add air after the barium. Adding air distends the bowel and improves the quality of the X-ray picture; it also reduces the amount of radiation used for each X-ray exposure because less X-ray dosage is needed to go through air. This examination is then called an *air contrast barium enema.*

During the examination, the radiologist watches the colon on a television screen to monitor the colon's filling. Small spot films of any area of interest or concern in the colon are also taken at this time. When the colon is adequately filled with barium and air, the technologist takes overhead pictures of the entire colon from several angles and with the patient turned in different directions.

When the pictures have been taken and reviewed, the patient then goes to the bathroom to evacuate the barium and air. The patient may still feel distended afterwards and later that day, but there are usually no other aftereffects from the barium; it just passes out in small amounts over the next few days. Some people find the barium constipating, but eating normally and drinking plenty of liquids usually prevents this problem from occurring.

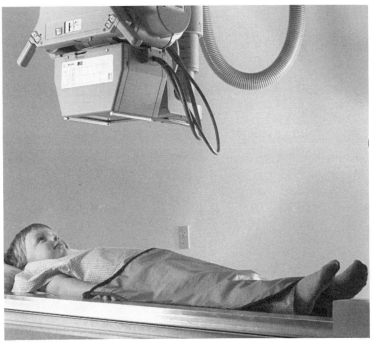

Child ready for X-ray examination of the abdomen. Note lead apron shielding lower part of body. X-ray tube is over child and film is in table under child.

CHAPTER SEVEN
Other Imaging Procedures

Although X-rays are still the best way in which to "see" many parts of the body, newer types of examinations are now used for some areas of the body or for special problems. These examinations include ultrasound, isotope scanning, computerized tomography (CT) and magnetic resonance imaging (MRI).

Several different forms of imaging are used for these examinations: ultrasound uses sound waves; isotope scanning uses an injection of a small dose of radioactive material; CT uses cross-sectional X-rays; and MRI uses a combination of magnetic fields and radio frequencies. These examinations are sometimes used in place of conventional X-rays; they can also be used in combination with X-rays to provide additional or different types of information.

The choice of examination used depends on the nature of the problem, the area of concern, the local availability of the different types of examinations and, occasionally, cost considerations.

ULTRASOUND (ECHOGRAM OR SONOGRAM)

Ultrasound is a type of energy, but differs from X-ray, isotope scanning and other imaging procedures because it uses no ionizing or electromagnetic radiation. Ultrasound uses sound waves of a pitch well above the normal hearing range of humans or animals. Very high doses of ultrasound can damage tissue, just as radiation and other forms of energy can when used in excessive amounts. When ultrasound is used in small, controlled amounts, however, it can provide much valuable information.

Ultrasound for medical examinations is used for short periods of time and at low power levels. Safe levels for ultrasound have been established by the American Institute of Ultrasound in Medicine (AIUM), the professional and scientific organization concerned with ultrasound for medical purposes. When ultrasound is used at or below these levels, scientists have been unable to show any significant biological effects on human tissues.

During an ultrasound examination, the doctor or ultrasonographer (a person who has had special training in the use of ultrasound) places a hand-held transducer (a broad-tipped, smooth instrument) in contact with the skin over the area to be examined. A gel-like substance is used on the skin to improve contact, and the transducer is then gently moved back and forth across the area being examined.

The transducer is a combination of a transmitter and a receiver which sends and receives the ultrasound waves. A sound wave travels out from the transducer, and as it meets different tissues in the body, some of the sound is reflected by the tissue and returned to the transducer. (The reflected sound is

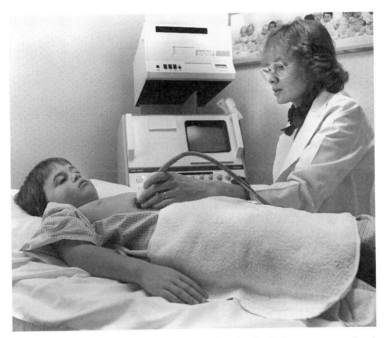

Ultrasound examination of child. Technologist (ultrasonographer) is holding probe on child's abdomen. Ultrasound picture (of the child's kidney) is displayed on monitor.

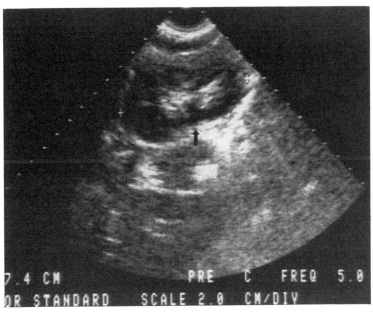

Ultrasound picture of a kidney (see arrow).

similar to an echo, and this is why the term "echo" has been used for this procedure.) An image is formed from the returning sound and is relayed to a television screen. This image is then photographed for further study (thus the term "sonogram," meaning a picture from sound). By looking at these images on the screen and in the photographs, a doctor can check the size, outline and inside structure of many organs.

Ultrasound is commonly used to examine a baby (fetus) for growth and development while in the mother's uterus. When ultrasound is used to examine a fetus, the doctor can determine the size, position and age of the fetus and check for abnormalities. After birth, ultrasound can be used to examine a baby's brain or abdomen for a tumor, bleeding or obstruction.

Congenital heart defects are also examined by ultrasound. The examination is called an *echocardiogram*. During this procedure, a doctor can examine the chambers of the heart and the main vessels entering and leaving it. This examination is now commonly used in place of an angiocardiogram.

Ultrasound is frequently used to examine the abdomen of a child in whom a tumor is suspected, and children who have frequent urinary tract infections often have an ultrasound examination of their kidneys. The gallbladder, liver and thyroid may also be examined by ultrasound.

Ultrasound is especially valuable in examining the area of the reproductive system because no radiation exposure is required. Ultrasound is often used for imaging the female pelvis, since the uterus and ovaries are readily examined. The male testes are also easily and safely examined by ultrasound.

Pelvic ultrasound may be used for girls who are going through puberty and who have menstrual problems while their bodies become adjusted to new levels of hormones. They may have pain during ovulation or during menstruation, and a pelvic ultrasound can often help determine whether or not there is a problem.

During a pelvic ultrasound examination, the bladder must be full, because ultrasound can "see" through fluid, but not air. The patient must drink 6 to 8 glasses of liquid before the examination. The examination itself is not painful, since the transducer (ultrasound probe) is moved over the abdomen with gentle pressure. There may be some discomfort because of the full bladder, however. An ultrasound examination outlines the uterus and ovaries, so that cysts and infections can be easily seen.

Ultrasound is also used to examine the male reproductive system. The testes are easily seen with ultrasound and can be examined for cysts, tumors, infections and trauma.

COMPUTERIZED TOMOGRAPHY (CT)

This examination is sometimes called a "CAT" scan. "CT" or "CAT" stands for *computerized tomography* or *computerized axial tomography*. The word "tomography" comes from the Greek and means a picture of a slice or section. The "axial" refers to the axis, or cross section, of the body that is seen on the X-ray.

During a CT examination, special detectors record the amount of X-rays passed through a very thin slice (or section) of the body. This information is then sent to a computer, which uses complex mathema-

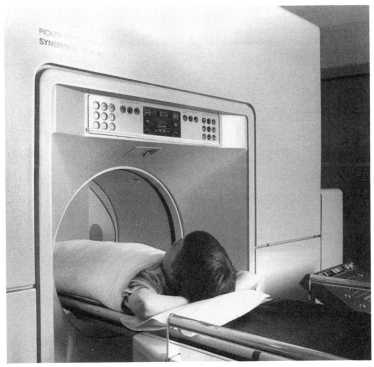

Child ready for CT examination of chest or abdomen. The part of the body being examined goes through the "ring" of the scanner.

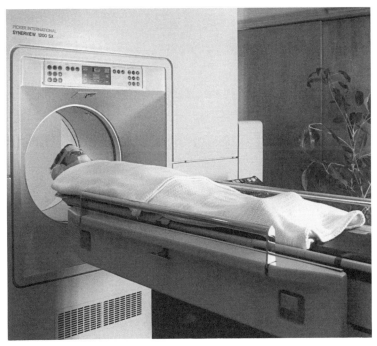

Child ready for CT examination of the head. Chin and forehead are lightly taped to help diminish motion of head during examination. The head is the "ring" of the scanner.

tical calculations to reconstruct the images almost instantly. The images show cross sections of the body like sections from an egg-slicer, with the X-rays doing the "slicing." The study is generally limited to one area of the body, such as the head, abdomen or pelvis.

The images from a CT scan are reproduced on a television-like screen and are then recorded on a special type of film used for recording video screen images. A CT scan provides doctors with a wealth of information that cannot be seen on other types of X-rays. The procedure takes longer (about 30 to 45 minutes) than plain X-rays because more pictures are taken.

A CT scanner is a large piece of equipment that has a "ring" in the middle of it. During the examination the patient lies on a table, which moves slowly into the ring while the X-rays are taken. The patient will feel no pain or discomfort, but it is often necessary to restrain small children to ensure that they do not move during the course of the examination. It may be necessary for the pediatrician to provide sedation for a very small child or infant. Many patients, however, relax enough to fall asleep while the CT scan is being done.

ISOTOPE SCAN

An isotope scan, also known as a nuclear scan, is usually performed in the nuclear medicine department of a hospital. The nuclear medicine department is usually part of the radiology department or is included under the more modern term, "imaging" department.

During an isotope scan, a doctor or nurse injects a small dose of a radioactive isotope, specific for a particular organ, into a vein. The isotope is allowed to accumulate in the target tissue for a specified period of time. The amount of time varies according to the part of the body being examined. The patient is then positioned in front of a camera, called a gamma camera, which records the radiation coming from the target tissue within the patient. The radiation recorded by the gamma camera forms an image or picture, which is then studied by the radiologist for abnormalities.

One of the most common scans is a bone scan, which is done when there is a possibility of a bone infection or tumor. A liver scan is performed in cases of injury, suspected tumors or congenital abnormalities. Thyroid scans are performed for suspected overactive or underactive thyroids, or for tumors. Kidney scans may be performed after an injury or to investigate the cause of high blood pressure.

The radioactive material that is used for these procedures gradually loses its radioactivity over time. For example, the most common isotope used (technetium) loses half its activity every 6 hours and continues to lose half of the remainder every 6 hours, until only a tiny, immeasurable fraction remains. The amount given is tiny to begin with, and the camera is very sensitive to these small amounts of radioactivity. Isotope examinations take from one to several hours, depending on how long the isotope takes to accumulate and how many views need to be taken.

During an isotope scan, the radiation from within the patient forms the image. In conventional X-ray examinations, the X-ray is the source of radiation which forms the image. The doses to the body are similar, although exact comparisons are difficult because of the differences in the examinations. For example, a bone scan, which is a very common examination, gives approximately the same dose to the body as a barium enema.

MAGNETIC RESONANCE IMAGING (MRI)

This procedure was previously called NMR, for nuclear magnetic resonance, but the word "nuclear" is often associated with negative connotations such as nuclear war, so MRI, or MR, was adopted as a better name for this procedure.

Magnetic resonance imaging is a completely different form of imaging from conventional X-rays, CT scanning or ultrasound. It uses a very strong magnetic field to line up the various atomic particles of which the body is composed. While the magnetic field is switched on, radio frequencies are also used to stimulate the atoms. When the atoms "relax" back to their normal state, they send out a signal from which an image is formed.

Current MRI examinations take about an hour, and patients have to stay completely inside the scanner during this time. Because of the noise in the scanner, patients may be given earplugs to wear during the examination.

There are many uses for MRI, especially for the detection of brain diseases such as multiple sclerosis, spinal cord tumors, and some congenital brain abnormalities and their complications. The uses for MRI are increasing all the time. But MRI does not and cannot substitute for CT and conventional X-rays for many examinations. An MRI examination is expensive and is only recommended if the team of imaging specialists thinks it is the best procedure in the circumstances.

Because of the addition of these newer procedures to the types of examinations radiologists perform today, the names of many hospital X-ray departments and radiologists' offices have been changed in recent years. Names such as "Imaging Center" or "Diagnostic Imaging Department" are now commonly used in place of "X-ray Department" or "X-Ray Office." Diagnostic imaging procedures are an important part of medical care today, and this name change reflects the addition of these new types of examinations.

CHAPTER EIGHT

Preparing Children For X-rays

The most common X-ray examinations, those of the chest or bones, require little or no advance preparation. Some children may be frightened by the large, unfamiliar equipment in an X-ray room, however, and a simple explanation is often helpful for reassurance, depending upon the child's level of understanding. The child needs to know about the large size of the X-ray "camera" and that it makes a buzz or beep as it takes the "picture." Parents should also stress how important it is to hold very still while the X-ray is being taken so that the picture will be sharp and clear.

Several books have been written about children in the hospital, and some of these books include a picture of a child having an X-ray. These pictures may be helpful in preparing a child for what to expect in an X-ray room. A list of some of these books is included in the bibliography.

When a small child must have X-rays, it may be necessary to restrain the child during the short amount of time needed to take the X-ray. Restraining is done in the best interest of the child and is necessary for the best pictures. As in photography, movement will blur the X-ray picture and may make a repeat X-ray necessary.

Children who weigh less than 30 lbs. often have their chest X-rays taken while held in the correct position in a Pigg-o-stat (named for its inventor, Jalmer Pigg, Sr.). This device is a strange-looking contraption that does an excellent job of holding a child safely and firmly in position, with the arms up out of the way (see photo). Children often cry for the short time they are restrained, but this inflates their lungs (just as a deep breath does in an adult) and contributes to a better X-ray picture.

For other examinations, such as those of the skull, wrist or foot, someone may have to hold a small child still and in the correct position for each X-ray view. This is usually the parent or a relative, but may be anyone who is willing and able, over the age of 18 and not pregnant.

Parents may be in the room during the examination or may be close by or watching through a window. Anyone in an X-ray room during an examination wears a lead apron. X-rays cannot go through lead, and lead shielding protects against any possible effects of the radiation on other parts of the body not being examined. Lead shielding or thick concrete is also used in the walls and sometimes in the ceiling and floor of X-ray rooms.

Lead shielding can sometimes be used on the patient too, depending on the examination. If a girl's abdomen is being examined, the ovaries are within the area being examined, and shielding them would interfere with the examination. But shielding can be used while examining a boy's abdomen, since the testes are outside the abdomen. If the knee or wrist

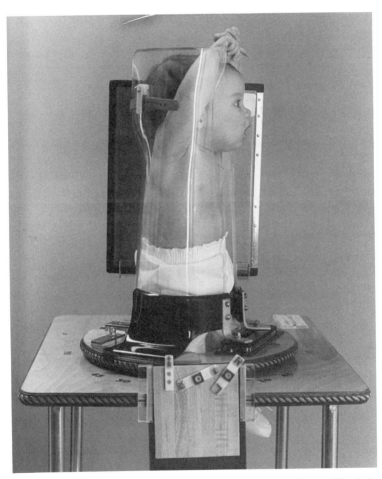

Infant in Pigg-o-stat, ready for X-rays to be taken. X-ray film is in cassette behind infant.

is being examined, an abdominal shield or apron can be used to protect the reproductive organs from any possible scatter radiation.

Remember, however, that the X-ray is directed only at the area in question. A chest X-ray does not expose the abdomen, nor does an abdominal X-ray expose the chest. There is no actual need for a shield, but there may be a little "scattered" radiation, and a lead shield prevents some of this radiation from reaching other parts of the body.

Children who undergo X-ray procedures and who are old enough to understand should be told in advance what to expect before and during an X-ray procedure. A child needs to know that for some examinations, he or she will have to change out of regular clothing and into a hospital-type gown with no snaps or metal on it. Snaps or metal objects will show up on an X-ray and may block out an area that needs to be seen.

A child must also be told about catheters or injections beforehand so that there is no surprise or confrontation at the time of the examination. This preparation makes it easier for everyone concerned.

Several X-ray procedures, however, do require some type of preparation on the day before or the day of the X-ray. Advance preparation for X-ray procedures varies with the examination. For an upper GI series, patients must fast overnight and eat or drink nothing in the morning so that the stomach is empty for the barium drink. A barium enema requires a little more preparation, since the whole colon (large intestine) must usually be emptied. A high volume of clear liquids and laxatives is needed for one or two days before the examination to achieve this emptying. A barium enema in a young child may not require any advance preparation at all.

Children do not need any preparation (other than an explanation of the procedure) for a voiding cystourethrogram (VCU). An intravenous pyelogram (IVP) requires fasting for several hours before the examination and a laxative for an older child. Patients have to fast for several hours before a CT scan where contrast is to be used; otherwise no preparation is needed. Nuclear scans and MRI require no advance preparation. Ultrasound requires no advance preparation other than a full bladder for pelvic examinations or fasting overnight for gallbladder examinations.

Most radiologists' offices provide written instructions for examinations that require advance preparation. Parents should not hesitate to call and request instructions if they are not provided by the referring doctor or the radiologist, or if there are any questions about the actual procedure.

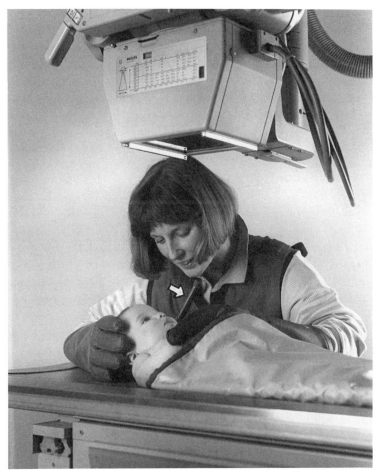

Mother holding infant in position for X-ray. Note lead apron and gloves on mother and radiation detector clipped to apron on mother (arrow). The detector measures radiation dose received by mother. This type of detector is required by law in some states.

CHAPTER NINE
Radiation Therapy

The use of radiation to treat diseases is called radiation therapy. Radiation therapy is almost always used to treat malignant diseases (cancer) and has saved or, at least, prolonged the lives of many cancer patients, both young and old.

One example of the successful use of radiation therapy is for Hodgkin's lymphoma. This is usually a disease of young people, and about 90% of those who receive radiation treatment are completely cured. Another example is a type of testicular cancer that affects young males. This cancer is also cured in more than 85% of patients who receive radiation.

Sometimes radiation is used to reduce the size of a tumor, and it may be combined with drug treatment (chemotherapy) and surgery for the treatment of a specific tumor. Radiation may also be used to treat the pain of terminal diseases.

The type of radiation used in radiation therapy is of a higher energy (shorter wavelength) than diagnostic X-rays and, of course, a much greater amount is used. Just as in diagnostic X-rays, however, the dose is carefully calculated and based on the type, size and location of the tumor and the size of the patient. The beam of radiation is even tailored and shaped to fit the tumor and the patient. For example, "mantle" radiation is a specially shaped radiation beam used for treatment of the chest in Hodgkin's disease to be sure as little as possible of the patient's otherwise healthy tissue is exposed.

When a child is diagnosed as having cancer, there are three basic treatment options:radiation therapy, chemotherapy and other medications, and surgery. The child's physician and a cancer specialist (oncologist) evaluate the situation, and a decision is then made about which type of treatment to use. The treatment may include one or more of the three types of therapy.

The decision to start radiation therapy is made by a team of doctors: pediatricians, surgeons, oncologists and radiation oncologists together. Then the child is evaluated in minute detail by a radiation therapist. Special measurements are made to assist in the detailed planning of the treatment, and a special X-ray machine called a simulator may also be used to help with the treatment plan.

Radiation therapy technologists and physicists work with the radiation therapist (the doctor) to determine exactly what machine settings, field sizes and treatment times will be used to give the correct radiation dose to treat this child's specific disease. The child may receive the first treatment on the same day the evaluation for therapy is done or within a few days.

Usually the treatments are given daily for several weeks. Although the initial set-up visit may take up to an hour or more, the regular treatments usually take less than a half hour once the child enters the treatment room.

Prior to actual treatment, the child may be asked to change into a hospital-type gown. Then he or she will go into the treatment room with the technologist, who helps position the child on the table. No one else is allowed in the room with the child during the treatment because of the much greater amount of radiation used in therapy than in diagnostic radiology.

The technologist will leave the room when the child is ready, close the door, and turn on the machine to begin the radiation treatment. The technologist will watch and listen to the child continuously by closed-circuit television. The room is also equipped with a two-way intercom so that the technologist can listen and speak to the child and give encouragement if needed.

It is very important that the child remain still during the time that the machine is turned on and the treatment is in progress. If necessary, special restraining devices may be used, and very young children may need some sedation.

The actual X-ray treatment cannot be seen, heard or felt, but the patient may be aware of some noises from the machine. The machine will usually be "on" for only a few minutes at most, but the technologists are prepared to switch it off immediately and come to the child if this becomes necessary for any reason. Once the initial routine is established, the treatments are quick and easy for most children to manage.

During the course of treatment, a doctor or nurse will usually speak to the parents and child on a regular basis. Any changes or concerns about the child should be reported immediately, in case there are changes that might require a modification of the treatment plan. The doctor will also examine the patient at regular intervals to check the progress of the treatment.

When the treatment is complete, the doctor will again examine the child and discuss any preliminary results with the parents. Radiation therapy often works gradually, with effects continuing after the regular treatments have ended. For this reason, periodic follow-up visits are scheduled.

Sometimes the total radiation dose can be divided up and given at different times to allow healthy tissue near the tumor to recover. Fortunately, malignant tissue is more sensitive to damage by radiation than is normal tissue, which recovers quickly.

Early temporary side effects of radiation therapy are some reddening and soreness of the skin (like a sunburn). Temporary hair loss may occur, but only if the head is in the area of the treatment. Other side effects may include tiredness or some nausea, but these, too, are temporary.

Years after radiation treatment, there may be an increased risk of malignancy resulting from the radiation therapy, but this is only a chance and not a definite aftereffect. This is a very acceptable risk for the many intervening years of life and health. Most cured patients, however, have no other problems and go on to live normal, healthy lives after radiation therapy.

CHAPTER TEN

New Developments and the Future of X-rays

Medical X-rays are becoming increasingly safe. Children who must have X-ray examinations today receive less radiation exposure than at any other time since the development of X-rays. New techniques, new cameras and machines and the use of video recorders all help to reduce the dose of radiation from an X-ray examination. Faster and more sensitive film, used in combination with modern intensifying screens, allows the exposure dose to be reduced 50 to 100 times below that which would be required for the same image without the screens. At the same time, the maximum possible information is obtained from each X-ray exposure. Research continues to improve techniques, equipment, film and screens so that each examination produces the optimal information while using the least radiation.

Doctors and other scientists continue to work toward reducing radiation exposure from X-ray procedures and to develop better and more accurate methods of diagnosing and treating illness. Procedures that do not use X-rays, such as ultrasound and magnetic resonance imaging, are being used more often. These examinations are sometimes used in combination with regular X-rays for additional information, but sometimes they can be substituted for an X-ray examination and provide the same information. The use of these procedures, where appropriate, also diminishes the total radiation dosage to the population as a whole.

Medical X-rays should never be used without good reason. But when they are needed for diagnosis or treatment, the risks of radiation exposure from X-ray examinations are minimal and far less than the risks from other everyday situations.

Parents need to be informed about the use of X-rays and other imaging procedures so that they can, in turn, explain their use in words that are appropriate for their child. The use of X-rays and other imaging procedures has made a valuable contribution to the quality of health care, and an understanding of their use can do much to assure continued good health for children and adults in the years to come.

CHAPTER ELEVEN

Mammography
A Special Message for Women

This discussion of X-rays and children provides an opportunity to include a special message for all women. Women should be aware of a very important X-ray called a mammogram, which is extremely important for the early detection of breast cancer. A mammogram can detect breast cancer in its early stages, when it is more than 90% curable.

A mammogram is a low-dose X-ray examination of the breast that can detect some cancers up to three years before a lump can be felt by even the most experienced examiner. Calcifications the size of grains of sand may be seen on a mammogram and could indicate an early stage of breast cancer long before it can be felt.

Breast cancer strikes one in every ten women in the United States and kills more than 40,000 women each year. It is one of the leading causes of death in women. Many of these deaths and much of the associated suffering experienced by the woman and her family can be avoided by early detection of breast cancer. Women who are over the age of 35 or who have a personal or family history of breast cancer should have a mammogram as a part of their regular physical examination.

During a mammogram, two X-ray views of each breast are taken while the breast is compressed between two flat pieces of firm plastic. Some women experience temporary discomfort while the breast is compressed, but the compression is necessary for the detection of the smallest cancers and also allows the use of the least amount of radiation.

The mammogram itself takes about 15 minutes, and the entire visit lasts about 30 to 45 minutes. The only preparation sometimes suggested may be to eliminate caffeine for several weeks prior to the examination. Caffeine sometimes causes breast tissue to become painful and lumpy, so eliminating caffeine may be recommended, especially for younger women.

Great emphasis has been placed recently on mammography of the highest quality for optimal detection of the smallest and earliest breast cancers. In previous years, mammography was performed with the regular X-ray tube. In recent years, however, a dedicated mammography unit has been developed. This unit is an X-ray machine specifically designed and used only for mammograms. A dedicated mammography unit is used to perform the special examination of mammography more effectively, more accurately and with a lower radiation dose than the older non-dedicated units.

The amount of radiation required for a mammogram is less than the amount used for standard dental X-rays. Mammography is considered a safe procedure, and the benefits resulting from early detection of breast cancer far outweigh any potential risk.

A mammogram, like all X-ray procedures, should be done by a qualified technologist and interpreted by an experienced radiologist. The radiologist may also recommend an ultrasound examination after viewing the mammogram. If a lump is present or questioned, ultrasound is helpful in determining whether or not it is a cyst. Breast lumps are common, and most are benign (that is, they are not cancer). Many breast lumps are normal breast tissue (either fatty, glandular or fibrous), and some are cysts.

Breast pain is also relatively common and is not usually caused by cancer. Most breast pain is the result of glandular tissue responding to hormonal stimulation during the menstrual cycle. Although breast pain or lumps do not necessarily mean cancer, they should always be reported to a doctor.

Because of the importance of early detection of breast cancer, the American Cancer Society, The American College of Obstetricians and Gynecologists and the American College of Radiology recommend these guidelines for women:

Age	Recommendation
20	Monthly breast self-examination
20 - 40	Physical examination by a doctor every three years
35 - 40	Baseline mammogram
40 - 49	Physical examination every year Mammogram every one to two years (depending upon the type of breast tissue seen on previous mammograms, how lumpy the breasts feel, and any family history of breast cancer)
50	Mammogram every year

Bibliography

American Cancer Society, *Cancer Facts and Figures-1988*. New York, NY: American Cancer Society, 1988.

Cohen, Bernard L. and I-Sing Lee, "A Catalog of Risks." *Health Physics*, June 1979, p. 721.

Committee on the Biological Effects of Ionizing Radiation, *The Effect on Populations of Exposure to Low Levels of Ionizing Radiation: 1980.* Washington, D.C.: National Academy Press, 1980.

National Council on Radiation Protection and Measurements, *Ionizing Radiation Exposure of the Population of the United States (Report No. 93).* Bethesda, MD: NCRP Publications, 1987.

FOR FURTHER READING

Hall, Eric J. *Radiation and Life*. New York: Pergamon Press, 1984

BOOKS FOR CHILDREN

Ray, H.A. *Curious George Goes to the Hospital.* Boston: Houghton Mufflin. 1966

Rockwell, Anne & Harlow. *The Emergency Room.* New York: MacMillion Publishing Company. 1985

Rogers, Fred. *Going to the Hospital.* New York: G.P. Putman's Sons. 1988.

Shay, Arthur. *What Happens When You Go to the Hospital.* Chicago: Henry Regnery Company. 1969.

Weber, Alfons. *Elizabeth Gets Well.* New York: Thomas V. Crowell Company. 1969.

Glossary

AIR CONTRAST   The use of air as well as barium to provide the contrast needed to outline the part of the body being examined. In the upper GI series, gas-forming crystals are given by mouth before the barium is swallowed. In the air contrast barium enema, the air is introduced with a small hand pump, after the barium.

ANGIOGRAM   An X-ray examination of blood vessels after the injection of contrast ("dye") into an artery or vein. An examination of arteries is also called an *arteriogram*. When veins are primarily being studied, the term *venogram* is used.

ANGIOCARDIOGRAM   An X-ray examination of the heart and surrounding blood vessels, performed after contrast has been injected into an artery or a vein.

ARTHROGRAM   An X-ray examination of a joint, most commonly the knee. Many other joints can also be examined, such as the elbow, hip and shoulder. Contrast material ("dye") and sometimes air are injected into the joint, and a series of X-rays are then taken.

ATOM   The basic unit of matter or the smallest particle of an element that can exist alone. Atoms of different elements are made up of various combinations of electrons, protons and neutrons.

BACK FLOW   See reflux.

BACKGROUND RADIATION   The radiation that is present in the earth and the atmosphere. We are all constantly exposed to background radiation. This type of radiation comes from the earth, the sun and the stars. The average background radiation to which the population of the United States is exposed is 100 millirems per year.

BARIUM   A natural substance which is mined and then processed into barium sulphate, the form used in X-ray examinations of the gastrointestinal (GI) tract or system. Like calcium and lead, barium absorbs most of an X-ray beam, and therefore makes the part of the body containing barium stand out sharply in contrast to surrounding structures. For an upper GI series, the barium is made into a liquid, often colored pink and strawberry flavored, giving it the consistency and appearance of a thick milkshake. For a barium enema, it is usually made into a white liquid.

BARIUM SWALLOW (OR ESOPHAGRAM)   An examination of the swallowing mechanism and the esophagus, which is the muscular tube leading from the mouth to the stomach. During the examination, a radiologist watches the patient's esophagus while he or she swallows barium.

BARIUM ENEMA   A barium examination of the colon, or large bowel, usually performed with barium and air. See "Air Contrast Barium Enema." The barium and air are introduced through a catheter, which is placed in the rectum. The colon is then filled to the point where the large and small bowel meet in the right lower abdomen, near the appendix.

CASSETTE   A hinged, light-tight holder for the

X-ray film. The film is sandwiched between two intensifying screens. The cassette with the film is placed behind the area of interest so that the X-ray, after passing through this area, forms an image on the film, which is then developed and viewed.

CATHETER A thin plastic or rubber tube used to introduce contrast material ("dye" or barium) into different body areas as required for various X-ray examinations.

CONGENITAL ABNORMALITY An abnormality which is present at birth.

CONTRAST MATERIAL Also known as "dye." Contrast materials are necessary to make certain areas of the body visible in contrast to the surrounding body tissues. Bone, because of its calcium content, has good "natural contrast." The kidneys and intestines do not. There are two common groups of contrast materials:the iodine-containing group, also called "iodine dyes," which are clear liquids, commonly used for IVP's, cystograms, arthrograms, and angiograms as well as many other examinations. Barium is the other major type of contrast material. It is used for gastrointestinal (GI) examinations. It is never injected into blood vessels.

CONTRAST REACTIONS Any foreign material, such as medicines and some foods, can cause an adverse reaction in the body. The reaction may be very mild, such as a rash or hives, but occasionally more severe reactions occur. Contrast materials are foreign to the body, just like other forms of medicine, and occasionally cause a reaction. Contrast reactions are very rare in children, and now there are newer materials ("non-ionic") available which have an even lower incidence of reactions. Barium very rarely causes any reaction.

COSMIC RADIATION The radiation coming from outer space, from the sun and the stars.

CT OR COMPUTERIZED TOMOGRAPHY Also know as CAT, or computerized axial tomography. A type of examination in which the X-rays are taken in cross-sectional "slices" of the part of the body being examined. See also "Tomography."

DEDICATED MAMMOGRAPHY UNIT An X-ray unit used exclusively for performing mammograms. A dedicated unit produces a superior image and also uses much less radiation than the older non-dedicated system.

DIAGNOSTIC IMAGING A broader term to describe more accurately the specialty of diagnostic radiology. This is the field of medicine devoted to making or helping to make diagnoses by the use of multiple imaging procedures such as X-rays, radioactive isotopes (nuclear scanning), ultrasound, CT and MRI.

DIAGNOSTIC X-RAYS The use of X-rays to help diagnose disease or injury. Distinct from therapeutic radiology, in which X-rays and gamma rays are used to treat diseases.

DIAGNOSTIC RADIOLOGY The field of medicine devoted to making diagnoses by the use of X-rays and other imaging procedures. See also "Diagnostic Imaging."

DOSE The quantity of radiation absorbed per unit of body mass. The skin dose is the easiest measurement to make, but it is considerably higher than the dose to the body tissue inside. A tissue or organ dose would be more accurate, but this is a more complicated measurement to make.

DYE   The common term for contrast material, or the iodine-containing clear fluid, used for the IVP, cystogram, arthrogram and angiogram. It is not a "dye" in the true sense of the word.

"ECHO"   See ultrasound.

ELECTROMAGNETIC RADIATION   The spectrum of electromagnetic energy containing a wide range of wavelengths and energy levels. These wavelengths range from very short, such as cosmic and X-rays with high energy levels, to very long, such as radio and electric waves, with very low energy levels. In between are radiant heat and visible light (See Chart, Pg. 3).

ELECTROMAGNETIC SPECTRUM   See "Electromagnetic Radiation."

ESOPHAGRAM   See "Barium Swallow."

FLUOROSCOPE   A machine consisting of an X-ray tube and a fluoroscopic screen. X-rays from the tube beneath, behind or in front of the patient pass through the part of the body being examined and produce an image on the fluoroscopic screen.

FLUOROSCOPY   An examination performed with the use of a fluoroscope. The most common examinations are the upper GI series and barium enema. When X-rays strike a fluorescent screen, an image is produced. This image is intensified and transferred to a television monitor for real-time viewing. This is fluoroscopy. Spot films are also taken at this time.

GAMMA CAMERA   Used in nuclear medicine to detect the radiation coming from the radioactive isotopes which have been introduced into the body for the nuclear scan. The radiation coming from the isotope in the body is in the form of gamma rays, which are shorter than medical X-rays in the electromagnetic spectrum (See Page 3). Common examinations are bone, liver and kidney scans.

GI (GASTROINTESTINAL) SERIES   An examination of the GI tract. The upper GI series examines the esophagus, stomach and duodenum; the small bowel series examines the small intestine; the barium enema examines the large bowel.

GRAY   The international unit of radiation dose now being used to replace the rad. One Gray is equivalent to 100 rads.

INFRARED   Radiation on the long side of visible light (see diagram of electromagnetic spectrum on Page 3). Infrared radiation is radiant heat, like that from the sun.

INTENSIFYING SCREENS   Fluorescent screens used to intensify the effect of X-rays, so that the image is sharper and less radiation is needed to make the image. The fluorescent or intensifying screens are mounted on the inner surface of the hinged cassette, with the film sandwiched between them. Special crystals in the screen give off light (fluorescence) when stimulated by the X-ray beam. This enhances the image formed by the X-ray alone.

IONIZING RADIATION   The type of radiation which is capable of forming ions. Examples are X-rays and gamma rays, alpha and beta particles, electrons, neutrons, protons and other nuclear particles, but not sound or radio waves or visible, infrared or ultraviolet light. Ultrasound is not a form of ionizing radiation, nor is MRI.

IONS Atoms carrying a positive or negative electric charge resulting from the loss or gain of one or more electrons.

ISOTOPE Natural substances (elements) have several different physical forms. These are called isotopes of the element. They have the same chemical behavior, but different physical properties. This allows a radioactive form of a substance (like iodine) to be substituted for the natural form in the body. The radioactive isotope can then be detected and scanned by a gamma camera to form an image.

ISOTOPE SCAN An imaging procedure using radioactive isotopes of a naturally occurring substance. The isotope is injected into the body and goes to the "target" area. Radiation from the isotope is detected by a gamma camera, where an image is formed and then transferred to film. Examples are bone, liver and renal (kidney) scans.

IVP Intravenous pyelogram. Also known as IVU, or intravenous urogram. Contrast material ("dye") is injected into a vein, and as it flows in the bloodstream and is filtered through the kidneys, the urinary system is outlined by the "dye"; hence urogram. The word pyelogram is a more anatomic definition of the collecting system of the kidney. The examination always includes the kidneys, ureters and bladder.

MAGNETIC RESONANCE IMAGING OR MRI Previously NMR. Refers to imaging which uses a strong magnetic field to align the various atomic particles in the body. Radio frequencies are also applied at the same time. When the atoms "relax" back to their normal state, a signal is sent out, from which an image is produced. No X-rays are used for this examination.

MAMMOGRAM   An X-ray examination of the breast.

MICROWAVES   Another form of energy from the electromagnetic spectrum. Microwaves are a non-ionizing form of radiation.

MILLIREM   One thousandth of a rem (.001 rem). See also Sievert.

MOLECULE   A combination of one or more atoms; the smallest portion of a substance that has all the properties of the substance. An example is water: 2 atoms of hydrogen and one atom of oxygen make one molecule of water, or H_2O.

NUCLEAR SCAN   See isotope scan.

ONCOLOGIST   A doctor who specializes in the diagnosis and treatment of cancer.

OVERHEAD FILMS   The large format X-ray films taken with an "overhead" tube after a fluoroscopic examination of the upper GI tract or colon.

POLONIUM   Polonium 210 is a radioactive substance given off during the burning of tobacco. It is thought to be a factor in the development of lung cancer from smoking.

RAD   Stands for radiation absorbed dose. See also Gray.

RADIATION   Any of the many forms of energy listed in the electromagnetic spectrum. All are considered to have a wave configuration. Some are ionizing, and these have a higher energy and a shorter wavelength than the non-ionizing forms.

RADIATION ONCOLOGIST   Same as radiation therapist.

RADIATION THERAPIST   A doctor who specializes in the use of radiation to treat cancer.

RADIATION THERAPY   See Therapeutic Radiation.

RADIO WAVES   A form of energy with long waves. See "Electromagnetic Spectrum."

RADIOACTIVE ISOTOPE   An isotope of an element which emits radiation.

RADIOACTIVE MATERIALS   All materials that are a source of ionizing radiation.

RADIOLOGIC TECHNOLOGIST (R.T.) OR RADIOGRAPHER   A person who is specially trained in the use of diagnostic X-rays and X-ray procedures. In some states, radiologic technologists are required to pass a licensing examination certifying their competence in diagnostic radiological techniques.

RADIOLOGIST   A doctor who has received an additional three or more years of education and training in the use of X-rays and other imaging procedures for medical purposes.

RADON   A colorless, odorless radioactive gas which results from the decay of uranium, a radioactive material present in variable quantities in the earth's crust.

REFLUX   Reverse or back flow, usually referring

to backflow from the stomach into the esophagus or from the bladder into the ureter.

REM   A measure of the dose of any ionizing radiation to body tissue in terms of its estimated biological effect. See also Sievert.

SIEVERT   The international unit to replace the rem. One Sievert is equivalent to 100 rems.

SCATTERED RADIATION   Small particles of X-rays that are deflected in many different directions when X-rays pass through tissue.

SPOT FILMS   The small format X-ray films taken under fluoroscopic control. Usually combined with overhead films for the complete examination.

THERAPEUTIC RADIATION (RADIATION THERAPY) The use of radiation in the treatment of diseases, nowadays almost exclusively cancer.

TOMOGRAPHY   From the Greek word meaning slice. A tomogram is an X-ray of a "slice" or section of tissue. A tomogram, or a CAT scan, is done to examine in detail an area deep in the body, such as the kidney or the center of the lungs.

TRANSDUCER   A broad-tipped rubber or plastic topped probe or instrument used to make contact with the skin during an ultrasound examination. The transducer acts as a combination of speaker and microphone, both sending and receiving the ultrasound waves used to form the image.

ULTRASOUND   Sound waves which are of a much shorter wavelength and higher frequency than audible sound. By definition, ultrasound has a frequency of more than 20,000 cycles per second.

Diagnostic ultrasound commonly uses frequencies from 3 - 10 million cycles per second (3 - 10 megahertz). Ultrasound imaging can be used for diagnosis, but also has many other uses, such as in physical therapy (heat or massage).

ULTRAVIOLET A type of radiation on the shorter side of visible light in the electromagnetic spectrum which can produce a tanning effect on the skin. Ultraviolet as well as infrared radiation is present in the sun's rays.

URETHRA The channel between the bladder and the skin, through which the urine passes out from the bladder. It is quite short in girls and longer in boys.

VCU Voiding cystourethrogram. An examination of the bladder (cystogram) and the urethra, usually performed because of frequent urinary tract infections.

WAVE LENGTH The distance between the peaks or troughs of two consecutive waves (See illustration on Page 3).

X-RAY FILM Special high-speed film which is affected by X-rays to form an image on the film. The effect is similar to that of visible light on photographic film. The average speed of X-ray film used with modern intensifying screens in diagnostic examinations is over 1000. The film, when processed by development and fixation processes, produces the X-ray image.

X-RAY IMAGE Because of the differential absorption of X-rays as they pass through different body tissues, an image is formed on film. This causes varying degrees of blackening, depending upon how much of the X-ray has been absorbed and how much reaches the film. The X-ray image which results is a two-dimensional image of a three-dimensional structure.

X-RAY (ROENTGEN RAY) A form of electro-magnetic radiation with high energy and short wavelength formed by the sudden stopping of high speed electrons. X-rays are capable of penetrating tissues and objects to a varying degree, depending on their composition.

X-RAY TUBE A glass tube containing two electrodes, the cathode (negative) and the anode (positive), in a vacuum. A high voltage current sends high speed electrodes from cathode to anode, where they strike a metal target, thus producing X-rays.

Index

A

B

C

D

E

F

G

H

I

K

L

M

S

T

X

X-ray film   24, 28, 95, 103
X-ray image   12, 23, 28, 103, 104
X-ray tube   24, 50, 88, 97, 104
X-rays   1, 2, 5, 6, 9-13, 17, 18, 20-24, 28, 31, 33, 35,
         36, 41-43, 45, 46, 49, 57, 64, 69, 71, 73, 74,
                   82, 85-88, 93, 96-98, 100-104

Notes

YOUR CHILD AND X-RAYS
A Parent's Guide to Radiation, X-rays and Other Imaging Procedures

Avice M. O'Connell, M. D.
and Norma Leonardi Leone

Additional copies of this book may be
ordered directly from the publisher.

To order, fill out the form below and send to:

Lion Press
P. O. Box 92541
Rochester, NY 14692

Other Books Available From Lion Press:

A Mother's Guide To Computers $ 5.95

From Nonnie's Italian Kitchen $ 8.95

Please send _____ copies of Your Child and X-rays $8.95

_____ copies of A Mother's Guide
To Computers $5.95

_____ copies of From Nonnie's
Italian Kitchen $8.95

Enclosed is _____ for books plus $1.50 for shipping for the
first book and 50 cents for each additional book (New York
State residents add 7% tax).

Please type or print clearly:

NAME: _____

ADDRESS: _____

CITY: _____

STATE: _____ ZIP: _____